ASTHMA EXPLAINED

GW00544994

ASTHMA EXPLAINED

Graeme P Currie MBChB DCH MRCP(UK) MD
Specialist Registrar in Respiratory Medicine
Aberdeen Royal Infirmary

ALTMAN

Published by Altman Publishing Ltd, 7 Ash Copse, Bricket Wood, St Albans, Hertfordshire AL2 3YA, England

First edition 2004

© 2004 Graeme P Currie

The rights of Graeme P Currie to be identified as the Author of this Work have been asserted by him in accordance with the Copyright, Designs and Patents Act 1988.

Typeset in 10/12.5 Optima by Scribe Design, Gillingham, Kent
Printed in Great Britain by Ingersoll Printers Ltd, Wembley

ISBN 1 86036 028 9

All rights reserved. No part of this publication may be reproduced, stored in a retrieval system or transmitted in any form or by any means, electronic, mechanical, photocopying, recording or otherwise, without the prior written permission of the publisher. Applications for permission should be addressed to the publisher at the address printed on this page.

The publisher makes no representation, express or implied, with regard to the accuracy of the information contained in this book and cannot accept any legal responsibility or liability for any errors or omissions that may be made.

A catalogue record for this book has been applied for

COMMUNITY INFORMATION LIBRARIES	
H503413590	
Bertrams	27.05.05
616.238	£6.99

∞ Printed on acid-free text paper, manufactured in accordance with ANSI/NISO Z39.48-1992 (Permanence of Paper)

CONTENTS

ABOUT THE AUTHOR

Graeme P Currie MBChB DCH MRCP(UK) MD is a Specialist Registrar in Respiratory Medicine at Aberdeen Royal Infirmary and manages patients with asthma on a daily basis. He has completed a full-time 2-year research period investigating the effects of inhaled and oral drug treatment used in asthma and has published many articles in both European and American journals on different aspects of asthma management.

PREFACE

Asthma is an important and common worldwide condition affecting both children and adults. If undertreated, patients may suffer needlessly and uncontrolled symptoms may in turn severely impair their quality of life. It is therefore imperative that everyone with asthma, and those who care for someone with asthma, understand what the condition is, and are aware of the signs of less well controlled asthma, what treatments are available and the goals of such treatment. This book serves to provide readable and basic information about asthma. It is not meant as a substitute for seeking medical advice and speaking to health-care professionals, but as a means in which to consolidate pre-existing or expand upon scanty knowledge and reduce the burden of asthma in the community at large.

ACKNOWLEDGEMENTS

The Publishers would like to express their thanks to the following companies for allowing us to use photographs of some of their products: AstraZeneca UK Ltd (Turbohaler), GlaxoSmithKline (Accuhaler; Diskhaler), IVAX Pharmaceuticals UK (Autohaler), Neolab Ltd (Neohaler), and Schering-Plough Ltd (Twisthaler).

1 INTRODUCTION

Asthma is a common condition affecting roughly 10% of the adult population and 15% of children. For example, it is estimated that 5 million people in the United Kingdom are being treated for asthma, while nearly 8 million have been diagnosed as having asthma at some stage of their life. It can present in early childhood as well as at any time during adulthood. Although asthma can occur at any age, it is particularly common in children and young adults, and is probably the most common chronic (long-lasting) disease found in this age group. At any age, the severity of asthma varies widely, although most cases tend to be mild-to-moderate in nature. The number of people with asthma in a given population varies from place to place and is determined according to many factors such as race, sex, country of residence and social class.

No single factor has been discovered to cause asthma. Indeed, no-one knows what the cause of asthma actually is, but environmental factors such as viruses, exposure to different allergens, being given antibiotics as an infant and numbers of siblings (brothers or sisters) have all been implicated in its development. Asthma tends to run in families, which suggests an inherited factor may also play a part.

The number of people dying from asthma has decreased in recent years, although as many as 1500 people of all ages (mostly elderly) die of asthma in the United Kingdom every year. It is known that people with life-threatening episodes of asthma often have risk factors which are readily preventable. These include inadequate or inappropriate treatment, poor adherence to treatment and a lack of understanding of their lung problem. This underlines the importance of patients with asthma and their carers having knowledge of their condition and knowing what to do when asthma becomes less well controlled. It is also imperative that patients are treated with the correct type of therapy.

The following aims of asthma treatment can generally be applied to most patients living in most countries around the world:

1

- prevention of troublesome symptoms during the day and night
- prevention of deterioration of asthma control
- maintenance of normal activity levels
- maintenance of normal or near-normal lung function
- provision of appropriate treatment while minimising the risk of unwanted effects
- satisfaction with the package of care provided.

To help achieve these goals, asthma management guidelines in the United Kingdom are frequently updated. These provide all doctors and nurses with the best available evidence and information on how to treat their patients. Unfortunately, there is no cure for asthma, but modern medicine and a greater public awareness of the condition has meant that many people have the potential to have no symptoms whatsoever.

2 WHAT IS ASTHMA?

Background

To understand what asthma actually is, it is important to be aware of the structure of the airway (Figure 2.1). Air (containing oxygen) is inhaled through the mouth and nose, and passes into the windpipe (trachea), which divides within the chest into smaller air passages (bronchi) on the

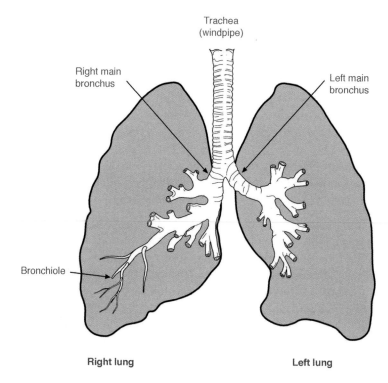

Figure 2.1   The structure of the airway.

left and right sides. The left passage further divides into two subdivisions, while the right one divides into three. These passages then subdivide even further into much smaller branches (bronchioles) which end in small air sacs (alveoli). It is in these air sacs that oxygen passes into the blood and waste gases such as carbon dioxide pass back into the airway and are exhaled by breathing out through the mouth and nose.

Asthma is characterised by three main abnormalities of the airway (Figure 2.2).

1 The first feature is inflammation of the inner lining of the airway. This extends from the larger air passages (bronchi) down to the tiny air sacs (alveoli), or in other words from the largest to the smallest airways. Experimental studies examining biopsy specimens of the airway of patients with asthma show the presence of higher than normal amounts of certain cells known as inflammatory cells. These cells are not present to any great extent in the airways of people who do not have asthma.

2 The second main feature is an increased 'twitchiness' of the airways, known as bronchial hyper-responsiveness. This means that the airways of people with asthma are more sensitive and more prone to narrowing compared to those of people without asthma.

3 Last, because the airways are prone to narrowing, the passage of air into the lungs is restricted, which is referred to as 'airflow obstruction'. This narrowing of the airways, or airflow obstruction, limits the flow of air in and out of the lungs. This in turn gives rise to symptoms such as wheeze and breathlessness.

It is important to point out that wheeze occurs in conditions other than asthma, as it is merely the sound produced from the passage of air through narrowed or obstructed airways. Airflow obstruction is usually intermittent and can reverse completely when medication is taken or when a susceptible trigger is no longer present. Since asthma is a condition that has a degree of reversibility, the patient experiences symptoms interspersed by symptom-free periods. In more advanced asthma that has been poorly treated, this narrowing of the airways (i.e. airflow obstruction) becomes fixed and the airways become permanently narrowed – a process termed airway remodelling. At this point, symptoms become more persistent.

4

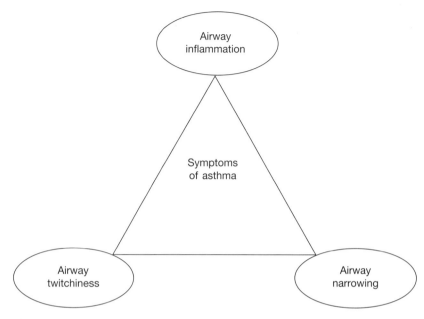

Figure 2.2   The three components causing symptoms of asthma.

Different types of asthma

There are several different types of asthma. For example, many patients develop symptoms on exposure to allergens, while others are termed non-allergic, which means that their asthma is not triggered to any great extent by allergies. Other patients have exercise-induced asthma, while those with occupational asthma develop symptoms due to the irritant nature of workplace triggers such as chemicals, fumes and dusts. Other types include aspirin-intolerant asthma (where the ingestion of aspirin causes symptoms) and cough-variant asthma (where cough is the predominant feature). Asthma can develop at any age and when it occurs in older people it is termed late-onset asthma. However, irrespective of the type of asthma, the treatment in terms of medication is very similar.

3 HOW ASTHMA AFFECTS PEOPLE

How does asthma affect people?

Having asthma should pose little or no limitation to normal domestic, social and working life. Many asthmatics continue to have symptoms unnecessarily because they either do not comply with their treatment or are taking the wrong type of treatment. In other words, if the appropriate medication is taken as prescribed, most asthmatics should have few or no symptoms most of the time. For example, sleep should be undisturbed and there should be very little or no limitation to the amount of exercise undertaken. Indeed, there are many famous sportsmen and women with asthma. However, a word of caution is that any asthmatic wishing to go underwater diving should request special advice from a doctor with expertise in this area as to whether this would be advisable.

How does asthma affect children?

Likewise, in children, if identified and treated appropriately, asthma should not cause any disruption to daily or school activities and exercise. It is, however, imperative that asthma is treated properly in childhood, as growth can sometimes be delayed in poorly controlled asthmatic children, resulting in a reduced height compared to children without asthma. Long-term scientific studies have generally shown that there is a far greater risk to a child's health from having poorly controlled asthma, than from taking a regular steroid inhaler to control asthma.

How does asthma affect pregnancy?

It is often quoted that asthma improves in one-third of pregnancies, remains the same in a third and worsens in another third. However, most women with well controlled asthma have normal pregnancies and go on to have normal deliveries with healthy babies. In women whose asthma is less well controlled, there is a higher risk of complications both for the mother and the baby. As a result, pregnant women with asthma need to be monitored closely and their treatment adjusted if necessary.

In general, the medicines used to treat asthma are safe in pregnancy, although specialist advice should be sought if uncertainty exists. Indeed, the risk of undertreated asthma to both mother and baby greatly outweighs the risk of any harmful effects arising from drugs. For example, blue reliever inhalers are considered safe in pregnancy, as are inhaled and oral steroids. Women with asthma should be encouraged to breastfeed. It is important to note that children of mothers with asthma are more likely to develop allergies than those mothers who do not have asthma. This risk may be reduced with breastfeeding. Furthermore, most medicines used to treat asthma are considered safe while breastfeeding.

4 THE IDEAL CONSULTATION – WHAT DOES THE DOCTOR/ NURSE NEED TO KNOW?

Medical history

Asthma is relatively easy to diagnose from the history (what the patient tells the doctor), but sometimes if it is very mild it can be less obvious. There is no specific blood test, x-ray or biopsy that is routinely carried out to make a diagnosis. Usually the diagnosis can be made by speaking to the patient, with parents of a child, or with carers. If a doctor wants to find out if you have asthma he will ask you a variety of questions such as:

- Do you wheeze or get breathless easily?
- Do you have a cough?
- Do you suffer from chest tightness?
- When are your symptoms worse?
- Do your symptoms come and go?
- What brings on your symptoms?
- Do you have hay fever or eczema?
- Do you have any allergies?
- What medication do you take?
- Do you smoke?
- Are your symptoms worse at work?
- Is there a family history of asthma?

The answers to these questions will help the doctor decide whether or not you are likely to have asthma. For example, patients may complain of symptoms, such as chest tightness, wheezing and breathlessness, being worse overnight and in the morning, with fewer problems in the afternoon and evening. However, often the only complaint is an irritating nonproductive cough which may be especially troublesome at night. This is particularly common among children and it is easy for all concerned to wrongly put this down to recurring colds or chest infections.

It is common for asthmatics to have another family member already diagnosed as being asthmatic, or they may have another allergic disease such as hay fever (allergic rhinitis) or eczema (dermatitis). It is also important to be aware of possible trigger factors such as pollen, infections, pets, feathered and furry animals, chemicals, environmental toxins, cigarette smoke and exercise. Other people with asthma develop symptoms on ingestion of aspirin or drugs with a similar chemical composition, known as non-steroidal anti-inflammatory drugs; common examples include ibuprofen (Brufen) and diclofenac (Voltarol). Another class of drug that often precipitates symptoms are beta-blockers. These are taken in tablet form and used for control of blood pressure, angina and prevention of a heart attack, but can be also found in eye drops used to treat glaucoma. However, before thinking about discontinuing these drugs, it is important to consult your doctor as to whether this would be advisable. It is also important to tell your pharmacist that you have asthma, as many over-the-counter medications can aggravate it.

Examination

Patients with asthma often do not have anything abnormal to find when examined, but sometimes there will be evidence of other allergic diseases such as the skin rash of eczema or reddened watery eyes or runny nose suggestive of hay fever. During an episode when the condition is at its worst, patients may have a wheeze which the doctor can hear with his stethoscope; in more severe cases a wheeze can be heard coming from the mouth.

Examining the heart and lungs may also help in excluding other diagnoses which cause breathlessness. In some patients, the doctor may want to arrange further investigations.

5 HOW IS IT DIAGNOSED?

Adults

Usually the doctor will be able to tell you if you have asthma by taking the history and performing an examination as outlined in Chapter 4. Sometimes the doctor may give you a peak flow meter to use, which measures the rate at which you can breathe out (Figure 5.1). Patients with narrowed airways often have a reduced peak flow, especially in the mornings or when exposed to an asthma trigger. If, however, the peak flow results are normal when the patient has symptoms, then it is less likely that the patient has asthma. Serial peak flow measurements are also a useful way of monitoring how well asthma is being controlled by treatment (Figure 5.2).

To use a peak flow meter properly you should:
* set the pointer to zero
* take a deep breath in
* seal your lips around the mouthpiece
* blow out as hard and fast as you can
* record the number next to the pointer.

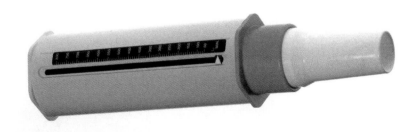

Figure 5.1   Peak flow meter.

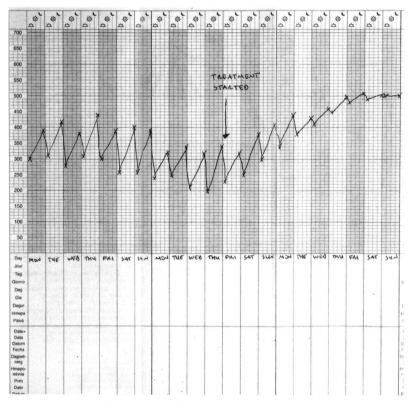

Figure 5.2 Variability in peak flow readings in a patient with asthma, and reduction in variability and improvement in peak flow after starting treatment.

The blows should be taken first thing in the morning, last thing in the evening and sometimes in between these times on advice of the doctor. Only the best of three attempts should be recorded into the peak flow diary. A 20% difference in peak flow during three consecutive days is generally regarded as being highly suggestive of asthma. It is usually necessary to monitor the peak flow for a couple of weeks to gain an overall picture.

A chest x-ray, especially if the patient smokes, may also be performed but this is not essential. This can be useful in excluding other causes of breathlessness and wheezing. Sometimes if the doctor is uncertain whether asthma is the diagnosis, patients may be referred to hospital for more specialised breathing tests or may be given an appointment with a hospital doctor specialising in asthma. Last, if the doctor suspects that your asthma is triggered by specific allergies, he may arrange for skin allergy tests to be carried out in hospital or he may arrange an allergy blood test.

Children

In young children, making the diagnosis can be a little more difficult, although the basic principles are similar to establishing the diagnosis in an adult. The likelihood of asthma being present is increased if there is already a history of it or of allergies in the family. Particular features that might alert the doctor or nurse to consider the diagnosis of asthma in a child include symptoms especially after exercise, inability to keep up with friends during sports or a persistent cough. If there are other associated features such as cough with thick green sputum, failure of a child to grow well, excessive vomiting or breathing problems present from an early age, the doctor should be alerted that there may be something else wrong. Referral to a hospital child specialist (paediatrician) may then be warranted.

Occupational asthma

Up to 10% of all asthma may be caused by exposure to substances such as chemicals and dusts at work. For example, some people may find that they are better at weekends or when on holiday, with symptoms prominent only in the workplace. However, it is important to be aware that many people are more active at work than at home, which may therefore be the reason for work-related symptoms. To be more certain of the diagnosis of occupational asthma, it is helpful to record the peak flow when at work and compare this to values when not at work. However, before an individual considers alternative employment or workplace environment, the diagnosis should usually be confirmed and discussed with a specialist.

6 KEEPING CONTROL OF ASTHMA

It is important to be aware that most asthma is classed as being mild-to-moderate in nature and can be relatively easily controlled with appropriate medication. However, despite a greater knowledge of the underlying disease process, better treatment and more widely adopted treatment programmes, asthma remains a common cause of hospital admission, ill health and, very rarely, death. It is noteworthy that in the United Kingdom there are a greater number of deaths in young people in the summer months, while in winter more older people die of asthma. Many fatal and near-fatal episodes of asthma are associated with problems that may be avoidable such as:

- failure to take prescribed medication
- alcohol or drug abuse
- failure to take advice from doctors
- being overweight
- self-discharge from hospital
- social isolation
- psychiatric illness
- inability to accept the diagnosis (denial)
- lack of understanding of asthma
- domestic and marital problems
- employment and income problems.

Factors suggesting asthma is not ideally controlled

Asthma tends to be a variable disorder and patients should be aware that they are prone to develop more or fewer symptoms at one point or another. When asthma is becoming less well controlled, it can be recognised relatively easily by both carers and patients. For example, increasing symptoms of chest tightness, wheezing and breathlessness

15

(especially at night-time), fall in peak flow readings, greater variability of peak flow readings (i.e. greater difference between morning and evening values) and increased reliever inhaler use, all indicate deteriorating asthma control. Using more than 2–3 puffs of reliever (blue) inhaler each day also suggests that asthma is less well controlled.

What should be done when asthma is less well controlled?

Many asthmatic patients have written action plans, detailing what should be done when asthma becomes less well controlled. Indeed, national guidelines on asthma treatment suggest that a written asthma action plan is an important part in its routine management. In particular, they have been shown to be an effective means of reducing the number of exacerbations and days missed from school and work. A written asthma action plan also means that patients are in control of their asthma, rather than being controlled by it.

During a cold or chest infection, or even for no obvious reason, asthma may become less well controlled. If a low-dose inhaled steroid is being taken at that time, the steroid dose should generally be increased. For example, if a patient is taking one puff twice daily of a particular steroid, it can be increased to two puffs twice daily during the less well controlled period. This rationale can also be applied to some patients using a particular combination inhaler (see Chapter 7). If these alterations to treatment prove unsuccessful and the patient fails to improve, medical advice should usually be obtained. Other more severe patients are instructed to use steroid tablets when their asthma becomes less well controlled.

Acute episodes of asthma

During an acute (abrupt) episode of asthma, the airways become more twitchy, especially during daily living activities which previously could be performed without difficulty. There is an increase in the number of cells of inflammation in the airway and also an increased amount of mucus secreted into the airway itself. The muscle around the airway contracts or tightens, which in turn reduces the diameter of the airway, resulting in obstruction to the flow of air.

16

This all results in frightening symptoms such as breathlessness, wheezing, inability to breathe in and out adequately and difficulty in speaking in sentences. Moreover, the patient's blue reliever inhaler may not help these symptoms. The pulse rate, breathing rate and blood pressure may also rise. In this situation, a doctor or an ambulance should be called immediately.

If you are admitted to hospital with asthma you will be given oxygen through a mask along with high-dose bronchodilators such as salbutamol (Ventolin), which opens up the airway. Often the salbutamol (Ventolin) will be given through a nebuliser (a machine designed to create a mist of drug particles which are easy to breathe in). You are also likely to be given oral steroid tablets, or steroids may initially be given as an injection straight into a vein. Most people respond to these measures, although a minority require additional medication or even transfer to a specialised medical treatment area for closer monitoring.

7 WHAT TREATMENTS ARE AVAILABLE?

With the availability of effective treatments, most patients with asthma will be able to lead perfectly normal and healthy lifestyles; only occasional review by a general practitioner or practice nurse is usually required. A small number of asthmatics will be less responsive to the treatment options available and will require closer monitoring from hospital specialists.

Smoking cessation

People who smoke have an accelerated decline in lung function. This is of even greater concern in asthmatics. Moreover, smoking or inhaling cigarette smoke from other smokers (passive smoking) irritates the airways, which in turn causes airway narrowing and symptoms. Parents who smoke increase the chances of their children developing wheezing-related illnesses. Smoking should therefore be strongly discouraged in everyone, especially in all asthmatics. Various measures are available to help individuals stop smoking. For instance, many general practitioners and hospitals run a smoking-cessation clinic. Nicotine replacement patches along with a tablet called Zyban (bupropion) can be useful in helping individuals who smoke more than 10 cigarettes a day. However, these measures are of little benefit without determination and a strong desire to stop.

Non-drug treatment

Drug treatment remains the mainstay of asthma treatment and reliance upon non-drug treatments is of limited benefit. There is no proven evidence that herbal medicines or homeopathy are of any great benefit in the control of asthma. Similarly, there is no scientific proof that acupuncture, hypnosis or the use of air ionisers confers any benefit. A special technique known as Buteyko has been devised with the

19

principle of reducing the rate of breathing. While it can be useful in asthmatic patients who over-breathe (hyperventilate), there is insufficient proof at present that its use can be applied successfully in a more widespread fashion.

Patients whose asthma is triggered by a known agent (or 'allergen'), are well advised to avoid that particular allergen, for example to avoid contact with dogs, cats, flowers or grass pollen. Some asthmatics find that decreasing the amount of house dust mite in the house by regular vacuuming, washing bed clothes at a high temperature or having wooden floors is of benefit. In order to optimise a healthy lifestyle irrespective of having asthma, most individuals should be encouraged to exercise regularly, lose weight if necessary and eat a healthy diet.

Drug treatment

Drug treatment is advised in most asthmatics in order to achieve the goals outlined in Chapter 1. Inhaled steroids, which are used to suppress

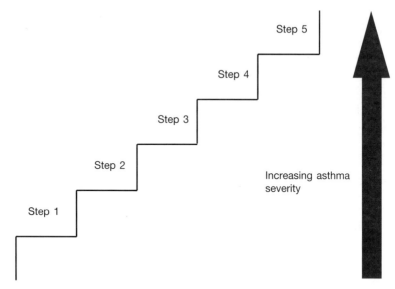

Figure 7.1   The stepwise approach to asthma treatment.

the airway inflammation, form the cornerstone of treatment in the majority of patients and require to be taken on a regular basis.

The over-riding principle of drug treatment is to eliminate symptoms at an early stage. Once control has been achieved, treatment should be increased or decreased according to both symptoms and lung function (in accordance with the variable nature of asthma). Patients should be encouraged to adjust their medication as part of an agreed action plan approved by their doctor or asthma nurse. To achieve good asthma control, guidelines suggest a stepwise (steps 1–5) approach to treatment (Figure 7.1): step 1 for very mild asthma, increasing to treatment used at step 5 for more severe asthma. Treatment, however, can be started at any step according to the severity of the asthma. It is important to note that all asthmatics are different, and sometimes treatment needs to be tailored to the individual patient. This in turn means that not all patients are treated strictly according to guidelines, but are treated in the way most suited for them.

Step 1 (relievers)

Inhalers used at step 1 are known as relievers and are used for instant relief of symptoms. These inhalers are called short-acting bronchodilators, or in other words, they open up (or dilate) the airway and allow rapid relief of symptoms. They exert their effects for only short periods of time – usually for 4–6 hours. Reliever inhalers should be taken at the onset of troublesome symptoms or 20–30 minutes prior to anticipated symptoms. These inhalers are usually blue in colour and common examples include salbutamol (Ventolin) and terbutaline (Bricanyl). They should be used without regular preventer treatment in only very mild asthmatics. Asthmatics requiring a reliever inhaler more than several times a week probably require preventer therapy, or in other words require to progress up the stepwise treatment escalator. A reliever inhaler should also be prescribed for most other patients for use 'if and when' they are breathless (in addition to regular preventer treatment).

Step 2 (preventers)

In anything other than the very mildest of asthma, preventer therapy should be used on a daily basis (Table 7.1). Low to moderate doses of inhaled steroid therapy (200–800 µg/day in adults and 200–400 µg/day in children) is introduced at step 2 of asthma guidelines to dampen down the airway inflammation and decrease the twitchiness of the airway. Steroid inhalers are produced by a variety of different manufacturers and therefore have different names; they are, however, generally brown in colour. It is imperative that any asthmatic who takes inhaled steroid therapy does so on a regular basis, as taking them intermittently confers no real benefit. Low-dose inhaled steroids are very safe to use even on a long-term basis, and constitute the mainstay of asthma treatment throughout the world. Compared to adults, the recommended dose of inhaled steroid in children is halved. In children, a reduction in the rate of growth, which can be associated with steroid tablets, does not appear to be of great concern with inhaled steroids. However, to be safe, monitoring a child's height should be carried out on a regular basis. It is important to point out that growth can be affected by poor asthma control to a greater extent than by medicines used to treat it.

Table 7.1 **Types of 'preventer' asthma treatment and common examples**

Inhaled steroid	Long-acting beta-2-agonist	Leukotriene receptor antagonist
Budesonide (Pulmicort) Beclomethasone (Becotide) Fluticasone (Flixotide)	Eformoterol (Oxis) Salmeterol (Serevent)	Montelukast (Singulair) Zafirlukast (Accolate)

Step 3

Some patients still have asthma-related symptoms despite taking low to moderate doses of inhaled steroids. Before altering treatment, the doctor or nurse should check that the patient is using the inhaler device properly and, just as important, ensure that the inhaler is actually being taken at all!

Guidelines suggest that the primary option at step 3 consists of adding in a long-acting bronchodilator (long-acting beta-2-agonist) to open up the airways. Long-acting beta-2-agonists dilate or open up the airway for a prolonged period of time (up to 12 hours) and also prevent the airway from narrowing. They should **always** be used along with an inhaled steroid.

22

Table 7.2   Combination inhalers and their constituents

Name of combination inhaler	Constituent (steroid and long-acting beta-2-agonist)
Symbicort	Budesonide (Pulmicort) + eformoterol (Oxis)
Seretide	Fluticasone (Flixotide) + salmeterol (Serevent)

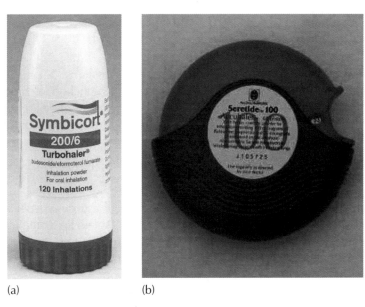

(a)   (b)

Figure 7.2   (a) Symbicort turbohaler and (b) Seretide accuhaler.

To make things easier for patients, these long-acting bronchodilator drugs can be combined with inhaled steroids in one inhaler (Table 7.2 and Figure 7.2). One such combination inhaler, budesonide/eformoterol (Symbicort; Figure 7.2a), can be adjusted (in terms of number of puffs) to match symptoms. It is therefore suited to fit in with written asthma action plans. Furthermore, Symbicort acts very quickly, which in turn may improve the patient's confidence, who may then be encouraged to use it on a regular basis.

If symptoms persist despite using a low dose of inhaled steroid plus long-acting beta-2-agonist, the dose of inhaled steroid can be increased to 800 µg/day in adults or 400 µg/day in children. Occasionally, some patients fail to gain benefit from the addition of an inhaled long-acting bronchodilator drug. In these individuals, it should be stopped and a drug in tablet form such as a leukotriene receptor antagonist or theophylline (see Chapter 8) should be tried along with the inhaled steroid.

Step 4

A minority of patients still have troublesome symptoms despite using regular inhaled steroids plus inhaled long-acting bronchodilator drugs. At this stage, there are several options. For example, the inhaled steroid dose can be increased, or a leukotriene receptor antagonist or theophylline can be added (see Chapter 8).

Step 5

Patients at this step are usually under the care of a hospital specialist. Many such patients are prescribed oral steroid tablets for continual or frequent use (see Chapter 8). Steroid tablets should be used on a regular basis with caution, especially in children. They can be associated with many side effects such as osteoporosis (thinning of the bones), slowing of growth in children, development of diabetes and cataracts, high blood pressure, weight gain and alterations in the immune system. It is important to be aware that in some patients steroid tablets are essential in the control of symptoms of asthma, and their benefits then outweigh the risks of side effects.

8 WHAT OTHER DRUGS ARE USED TO TREAT ASTHMA?

Leukotriene receptor antagonists

Important and useful drugs used in the management of asthma are called leukotriene receptor antagonists. They are usually well tolerated and do not have the troublesome side effects of steroid tablets. This type of preventer medication is sometimes used in patients who still have symptoms despite using regular inhaled steroids. Montelukast (Singulair) and zafirlukast (Accolate) are two examples commonly used in the United Kingdom. These drugs, which are taken as tablets, dampen down airway inflammation and open up the airway for a prolonged period of time (roughly 12–24 hours). They can be particularly useful in patients who are unable to take inhaled medication for whatever reason, for example in children and the elderly who may have difficulty in using inhalers. Montelukast (Singulair), which is taken once daily, is useful when taken alone in patients with exercise-induced asthma. It may also be effective in asthmatics who have hay fever or aspirin-sensitive asthma.

Theophyllines

A group of drugs called theophyllines (for example Uniphyllin Continus or Nuelin) are sometimes used in the management of asthma. They are generally used along with inhaled asthma treatments when symptoms persist. When taken at night, they can be particularly useful in controlling night-time symptoms. Similar to leukotriene receptor antagonists, they come in tablet form and are taken once or twice a day. Unfortunately side effects such as nausea, vomiting, abdominal pain and heart rhythm abnormalities limit their use in some patients. They also interact with many other drugs, which means that the doctor or pharmacist should check all other medications being taken before suggesting this type of drug. An injectable form of theophylline (aminophylline) is used to treat acute asthma in hospital.

Oral steroids

Steroid tablets (usually called prednisolone) are sometimes necessary when patients have an acute episode of asthma. Indeed, using oral steroids early at the onset of an exacerbation of asthma can reduce the need for hospital admission. Short courses (1–2 week duration) of steroid tablets are given to such patients, and tend to result in few worrying side effects. It is vitally important if anyone feels unwell while using oral steroids, or even after finishing a course, that they seek medical advice. Some patients with more severe asthma require long-term steroid tablets, which usually needs close monitoring by hospital specialists. Many patients feel far better in themselves when taking steroid tablets. However, it is imperative that they are only used if necessary, usually on the advice of a doctor or nurse.

Cromoglicates

These types of drugs are occasionally used in asthma and tend to be more useful in children, especially those with exercise-induced asthma. They are a form of inhaled medication and have little in the way of important side effects but can cause coughing. Common examples include sodium cromoglicate (Intal) and nedocromil sodium (Tilade).

Antihistamines

Antihistamines by themselves are of no use in the treatment of asthma. They are sometimes used (along with other asthma treatment) in patients who have a strong allergic component to their asthma; in particular, in patients who have hay fever and who suffer from troublesome allergies. Older antihistamines used to cause drowsiness, but more up-to-date versions do not cause this problem.

Anticholinergics

Inhalers containing this type of drug are sometimes used as reliever therapy in asthma. Occasionally patients are unable to tolerate salbutamol (Ventolin), and are given an inhaler containing terbutaline

(Atrovent) instead for rapid relief of symptoms. These drugs act in a similar fashion to salbutamol, but take a little longer to open up or dilate the airways. Sometimes this class of drug can be combined with salbutamol in a single inhaler or in a nebuliser.

9 INHALER DEVICES

Inhalers are used by most patients to deliver different types of medication to the lungs. Unfortunately, with all inhalers, a large proportion of the drug is deposited in the mouth and throat rather than in the lungs themselves. Before being prescribed an inhaler, it is important that the doctor or nurse demonstrates how to use it. The patient must then be able to use the inhaler device properly.

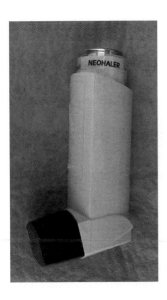

Figure 9.1   Metered dose inhaler.

One of the most common inhaler types is called a metered dose inhaler (abbreviated to MDI – see Figure 9.1). To use this device properly, the following instructions should be closely followed:

- Shake the canister.
- Take a full breath out.
- Put your lips around the mouthpiece.

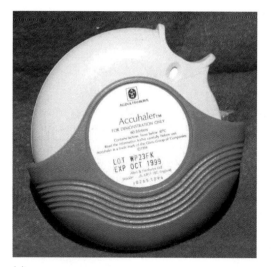

(a)

Figure 9.2 Different types of inhalers:
(a) Accuhaler;
(b) Autohaler;
(c) Diskhaler;
(d) Twisthaler;
(e) Turbohaler.

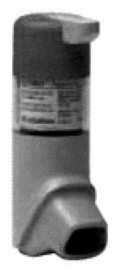

(b)

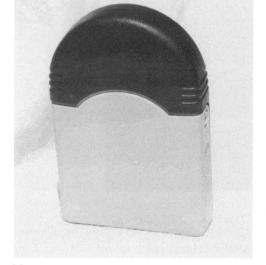

(c)

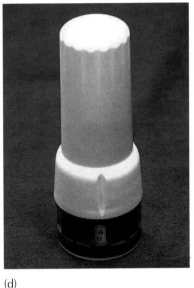
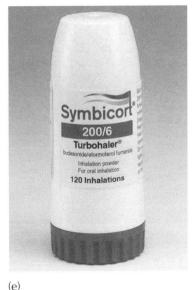

(d)   (e)

- Press only once with the inhaler in your mouth and at the same time suck inwards quickly.
- Hold your breath for up to 10 seconds.
- Breathe out normally.
- For a second dose, these steps should be repeated.

Many patients – especially children and the elderly – find difficulty in using MDIs and many other inhaler types are available. This has resulted in a bewildering array of different types of inhalers available for use. Common examples of different inhalers are shown in Figure 9.2. However, whichever inhaler type the patient finds easy to use and feels confident in using is a reasonable way of deciding which one is best. As a way of making MDI inhalers easier to use and to make them more effective, they can be used along with a spacer device (Figure 9.3).

How to use and maintain spacers

A spacer is a large plastic container with an opening at either end (Figure 9.3); one opening is to attach the inhaler and the other is a mouthpiece.

31

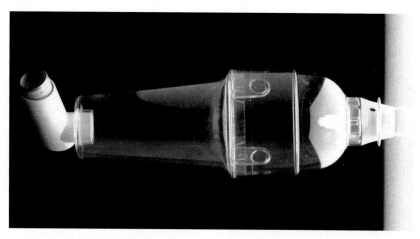

Figure 9.3   Spacer device plus metered dose inhaler.

Spacer devices have a chamber that receives the drug particles before they are inhaled. They serve two functions. First, they avoid problems in coordinating the timing of the inhaler actuation and inhalation and, second, they slow down the speed of delivery of the aerosol into the mouth so that less of the drug is deposited in the throat. Different manufacturers make different sizes of spacers and inhalers which should be used together. The following principles can be applied to most types:

- Make sure the inhaler fits snugly into the end of the spacer device.
- Take a full breath out and then put the spacer mouthpiece in your mouth.
- Press the inhaler (attached to the end of the spacer).
- Take a full breath inwards and hold your breath for up to 10 seconds if possible.
- Wipe clean the mouthpiece after use.
- Spacers should generally be cleaned at least once a month with soapy water and be left to drip dry.
- They should be replaced every 6–12 months, depending on the manufacturer's recommendations.

Inhalers for adults

An MDI plus spacer and another type of inhaler device called a dry powder inhaler (abbreviated to DPI) are the most effective hand-held devices – as long as they are used properly. Despite being useful in delivering drugs to the lung, the main disadvantage of spacers is that many people do not like the idea of carrying them around in view of their size. DPIs are breath activated, which means that coordination is less of a problem compared to using an MDI without a spacer. In other words, the act of 'sucking in' causes the drug particles to be released from the DPI, which are then inhaled. They are also less bulky than an MDI plus spacer and are more easily carried around. It is for this reason that many adults and children prefer breath-activated, hand-held devices (see Figure 9.2).

Inhalers for children (0–12 years)

Children under 5 years of age have difficulty using inhalers effectively by themselves. With the aid of a parent or carer, inhaled medication should be given using a spacer device to which an MDI is fitted at its end. In very young children, using a face mask attached to the other end of the spacer is helpful. In older children aged 5–12 years, an MDI plus spacer is as effective as any other hand-held inhaler – again provided it is used properly. Once at school, a spacer device may be too bulky and inconvenient to carry around. At this time, the doctor or nurse may decide to change to a DPI which is both easy to carry around and easy to use.

Nebulisers

Nebulisers are electrical powered machines which deliver high concentrations of a drug via a face mask. They create a mist of drug particles which is then inhaled by the patient. Nebulisers can be used during an acute episode of asthma, either at the patient's home, in an ambulance, or in hospital. Some patients with more severe asthma are given a nebuliser to use on a regular basis at home. However, it is important to point out that using a nebuliser is probably as effective as using an

MDI plus spacer correctly. Using a nebuliser can take as long as 10 minutes, while using an inhaler takes a fraction of this time.

10   COMMONLY ASKED QUESTIONS

Does stress cause asthma?

Stress and emotions do not cause asthma. In some people with established asthma, however, stressful situations can make asthma worse.

What are the side effects of inhaled steroids?

The two most common side effects of inhaled steroids are oral thrush (white plaques found on the tongue and inside of the mouth caused by a fungus) and an alteration in the quality of the voice. These are far more commonly found in patients taking high doses of inhaled steroids and can be minimised by brushing the teeth after using the steroid inhaler along with thorough mouth rinsing. In patients using a metered dose inhaler alone, using it along with a spacer device minimises this risk.

What are the side effects of long-acting beta-2-agonists (e.g. Serevent and Oxis)?

These drugs are usually well tolerated but occasionally people complain of palpitations (an increased awareness of the heart beating which may be faster or more erratic than usual) and tremor of the outstretched hand.

What are the side effects of leukotriene receptor antagonists (e.g. Singulair and zafirlukast)?

Leukotriene receptor antagonists have been shown to be very safe and very well tolerated. However, side effects such as rashes and abdominal pain have been reported.

What are the advantages of taking a combination inhaler?

First, it is easier to remember to take one inhaler rather than two. Second, the long-acting beta-2-agonist component [eformoterol (Oxis) or salmeterol (Serevent)] opens up the airways and keeps it open for up to 12 hours, while the inhaled steroid in the inhaler dampens the airway inflammation down. It is important to point out that eformoterol (Oxis) acts very quickly as well as being long-acting, which in turn gives patients fairly instant relief of symptoms.

How can I reduce the chances of my child getting asthma?

There is no reliable way of reducing the chance of asthma developing in a child. Some studies have suggested that breastfeeding reduces the chance of wheezing and development of asthma in children. The children of mothers who smoke have a greater chance of having wheezing-related chest illnesses than mothers who do not smoke. Furthermore, the cigarette smoke of parents can aggravate established asthma in a child.

Will my child grow out of their asthma?

Many children do grow out of their asthma, but there is no certain way of knowing who will or who won't.

Will I have to use inhalers for the rest of my life?

Many adult patients require treatment for asthma throughout their life and it is important not to stop taking inhalers without medical advice. However, it is generally advised that if asthma is well controlled over a period of 3–6 months, treatment can be cut back on the advice of the doctor or nurse.

What will happen if I don't take my prescribed inhaled steroid?

There will be a gradual build-up of inflammation in the lungs and you will feel progressively more breathless and wheezy. You will find that symptoms become resistant to the effects of salbutamol (Ventolin). Eventually you will probably require a high dose of inhaled steroids or a course of steroid tablets; you may even be admitted to hospital.

What is the difference between asthma and chronic bronchitis/emphysema?

Chronic bronchitis and emphysema tend to occur in smokers or ex-smokers. Their airways (unlike asthmatics) are generally permanently narrowed and respond far less well to inhalers. People with chronic bronchitis and emphysema often cough up discoloured sputum in the mornings.

Is there a greater risk of getting lung cancer if I have asthma?

No. There is no link between the two conditions.

Should I have a nebuliser at home?

Nebulisers should really only be used at home if advised by a hospital specialist, or occasionally by a general practitioner. If a patient uses a nebuliser at home without proper medical advice, they can become over-reliant on it. This means that there may be a delay before seeking specialist advice during a severe attack of asthma.

What precautions should I take when I go on holiday?

Most people with asthma can fly without any increased risk. It is impor-tant to have a reliever inhaler in hand luggage in the event of an asthma

episode while in an aeroplane. Some people who have frequent exacerbations of asthma find it worthwhile taking a course of steroid tablets
and antibiotics (prescribed by their doctor) on holiday with them in case
they run into problems while away. The vast majority of patients with
asthma do not require oxygen when flying. In patients with more severe
asthma, however, oxygen may be necessary, in which case it would be
advised by a hospital specialist. In flight, oxygen can usually be
arranged by contacting the particular airline.

11   CASE STUDIES

Case 1

David is a 19-year-old student with asthma who smokes two or three cigarettes a day. His elder brother and mother also have asthma. His general practitioner had previously prescribed him a steroid inhaler, but as he found no benefit from it after a couple of days he stopped taking it. For the past 6 months he needed to use his Ventolin (blue reliever inhaler) four to five times a day. He found this was fairly effective at reducing his wheezing and allowed him to play football twice a week. On one occasion, however, he was so breathless after football despite taking six puffs of Ventolin, he could not speak in sentences and felt his chest was tighter than it had ever been before. His friends were alarmed and took him to the local Accident and Emergency department.

Asthma explained

David has asthma and is using a reliever alone on a frequent basis. Unfortunately, he was not aware that steroid inhalers do not exert immediate beneficial effects. He also smokes. David clearly requires treatment for this acute severe episode, and the importance of using regular anti-inflammatory preventer therapy emphasised. It would also be important to discuss David's smoking with him and encourage him to stop.

David was treated in hospital with oxygen, Ventolin through a nebuliser and given steroid tablets to take for 10 days. Prior to being allowed home 2 days later, he was given an inhaled steroid inhaler (brown preventer) and instructed to use this on a twice daily basis, rinsing his mouth and brushing his teeth after doing so. He was also strongly encouraged to stop smoking.

Case 2

Kylie, who is aged 10 and not known to have asthma, is taken by her mother to see her general practitioner. Over the past 3 months she has noticed that Kylie is wheezy first thing in the morning and often has difficulty sleeping because of a 'barking' cough. These problems are worse when she has a cold. At present during the summer months, she has also been sneezing a lot, complaining of itchy eyes and a runny nose. Kylie had eczema as a younger child, which burnt itself out several years earlier. She has a cousin who uses a blue inhaler maybe once a week for asthma.

Asthma explained

Due to the uncontrolled inflammation, airway twitchiness and intermittently narrowed airways, Kylie has developed classical symptoms of asthma which are being made worse by colds and probably hay fever and allergies. She requires anti-inflammatory therapy to control this and something for her hay fever. There is a reasonable chance that she will grow out of her asthma. Kylie's general practitioner decides that she has allergic asthma and prescribes a steroid inhaler (brown preventer) to be taken twice a day, in addition to a blue reliever inhaler to be carried at all times to use 'if and when' she is breathless. He also decides that she has hay fever and a possible grass allergy, which may in turn be making her asthma worse. He prescribes her an antihistamine to be taken during the summer months, and gives her some antihistamine eye drops to relieve the grittiness which makes her constantly want to rub her eyes.

When seen for a follow-up appointment 2 months later, Kylie can sleep without coughing and no longer feels wheezy in the mornings. She also mentions that she can play a full netball match without having to rest two or three times during the game like she did before.

Case 3

Margaret, aged 58, who has never smoked, has had asthma for many years. For the past 8 years she has taken a low-dose steroid inhaler through a metered dose inhaler plus spacer device. Increasingly she has found herself waking up overnight coughing and at times struggling for a breath. She needs to use her Ventolin (blue reliever inhaler) usually once a night. She is becoming quite concerned about this as she feels irritable because of lack of sleep and her husband is beginning to complain because of being woken up every night.

Asthma explained

Margaret is taking a low-dose inhaled steroid (step 2 of asthma guidelines). Despite this, she still has symptoms suggestive of less well controlled asthma. Her general practitioner should consider altering her asthma treatment, as indicated by step 3 of current guidelines.

Margaret arranges an appointment with her general practitioner who first makes sure she is using her inhaler properly and confirms that she is, indeed, taking it as prescribed. Her doctor decides to prescribe a combination inhaler containing a higher steroid dose in addition to a long-acting beta-2-agonist. On review several months later, she has no symptoms whatsoever and even tends to forget that she has asthma. He decides to review her again in 3 months, and if she still has no problems with her asthma he plans to reduce her treatment.

12 USEFUL WEBSITES

Many patients with asthma have access to information regarding their condition from a variety of sources such as television, radio, books and magazines. Recently, people of all ages have gained access to the World Wide Web. Although this is an invaluable source of information, it is vital that the advice of doctors and nurses is taken in conjunction with advice gained from the internet. It is also important to know that often treatments advertised on the internet have not been tried and tested in rigorous drug trials, and may not be endorsed by your doctor. It is therefore imperative that any issues arising from access to the internet, involving even minor treatment changes, are discussed fully with a doctor. Three helpful and medically recognised websites are shown below:

* www.asthma.org.uk
* www.occupationalasthma.com
* www.asthma.org.uk/control

13 SOCIETIES, ASSOCIATIONS AND HELPLINES

Most doctors and nurses will be happy to pass on information about asthma, or will be able to direct you to someone who can. However, the following is a list of organisations that can provide further help, information and advice.

- National Asthma Campaign
  Providence House
  Providence Place
  London N1 0NT
  Telephone: 020 7226 2260

- National Asthma Campaign Scotland
  2A North Charlotte Street
  Edinburgh EH2 4HR
  Telephone: 0131 226 2544

- Asthma Helpline (open 9 a.m. to 7 p.m., Monday to Friday)
  Telephone: 0845 701 0203

- Smoking quitline
  Telephone: 0800 848 484 (Scotland)
  Telephone: 0800 002 200 (England)
  Telephone: 0345 697 500 (Wales)

INDEX

Note: page numbers in *italics* refer to figures and tables

complementary therapies 19–20
control of asthma *see* symptoms of
  asthma, control
cough 9, 40, 41
  persistent 13
cough-variant asthma 5
cromoglicates 26

deaths from asthma 1, 15
diagnosis 9, 11–13
diclofenac (Voltarol) 10
diet, healthy 20
Diskhaler *30*
diving, underwater 7
drugs *see* medicines
dusts, exposure to 5, 13

eczema 10
eformoterol (Oxis) 36
emphysema 37
examination of patient 5
exercise 7
  healthy lifestyle 20
  symptoms after 13
exercise-induced asthma 5, 25, 26

fatal episodes 15
flying 37–8

hay fever 10, 25, 26, 40
helplines 45
holidays 37–8
hospital admission 17
hospital referral 13
hyperventilation 20

ibuprofen (Brufen) 10
inhalation 3–4
inhalers 29, *30,* 31–34
  combination 16, 23, 26, 36, 41
  correct use 22
  dry powder 33
  metered dose 29, 31, 33
  preventers (brown) 21–2, 39, 40

relievers (blue) 8, 16, 17, 21, 39, 40
steroid 7, 8, 16, 20–4
  combination 36
  side effects 35
  stopping 37
  use 29
inheritance of asthma 1
Intal 26

late-onset asthma 5
leukotriene receptor antagonists *22,*
  25
  side effects 35
lifestyle, healthy 20
lung cancer 37

medical history 9–10
medicines 20–6
  asthma-inducing 5, 10
  interactions with other drugs 25
  over-the-counter 10
  safety in pregnancy 8
montelukast (Singulair) 25
  side effects 35

near-fatal episodes 15
nebulisers 17, 28, 33–34
  home use 37
nedocromil sodium (Tilade) 26
nicotine replacement patches 19
non-steroidal anti-inflammatory drugs
  (NSAIDs) 10
Nuelin 25

occupational asthma 5, 13
older people
  deaths from asthma 15
  inhalers 31
  late-onset asthma 5
organisations 45
over-breathing 20
Oxis 36
  side effects 35
oxygen administration 17